H[O]

BREATHE:

The Symptoms if You Get it Wrong, and How to Fix It.

by Sally Gething

Cold Hands and Feet; Pale Face and Skin; Difficulty in Catching Your Breath or Difficulty in Taking a Deep Breath; Asthma; Panic

Attacks; Hyperventilation Attacks; Allergies, Eczema, and Skin Conditions; Slack Jawline; Protruding Teeth; Elongated Face Shape; Dental Cavities; Repeated Chest and Throat Infections; Nasal Voice, Whispering Voice, and Losing One's Voice; Abnormal Breathing Patterns; Snoring; Sleep Apnoea; Lung Damage (including emphysema, C.O.P.D., Bronchiectasis); Hypertension/High Blood Pressure; and I.B.S (Irritable Bowel Syndrome).

ALSO BY THE AUTHOR

TOO LITTLE SALT: TEN ANNOYING SYMPTOMS

available in paperback

and eBook

CONTENTS

WELCOME

Hello and welcome. This is a book about breathing and how to do it correctly – it might not be as easy as it sounds! You should find the exercises easy to follow and you should start seeing positive results in the first few days. To get the best results I'd like you to read this book over five to ten days – or even longer if you wish. I'll take you through what you need to do, step-by-step. Within these pages you'll find lots of easy breathing and posture exercises (all done from the comfort of a chair - don't worry, you don't have to lie on the floor!), and all of them you will be able to do on your own, without anyone else looking at you, or judging how well you are doing.

Some of the exercises such as 'How to Breathe In and Out' and 'Don't Stretch' may sound simple, but they are all little parts of a whole. Just as in a car engine, where some parts –

like the oil cap - may seem minor, without them, the engine won't perform properly. It is the same with breathing. If you are doing a few little things wrong, then it can have a huge effect on your breathing, making it less effective and cause you a host of unpleasant and annoying symptoms.

This book contains a variety of breathing exercises interspersed with pockets of handy information. This means you can start on the exercises and practice them whilst moving on to the next chapter.

It's better if you don't try to do everything in one go. As I'm not there to watch you I'll ask you to assess how you are doing yourself, and if you have done enough that day, then have a rest, and come back to it in 24 hours. I may ask you to relax and to drop your shoulders too. Most people, when they are attempting new breathing exercises have a tendency to tense up and, because of this, their shoulders will creep up round their ears. Be aware if this happens to you – if it does, say to yourself: 'Relax, and drop your shoulders.' If you are in any doubt, then have a rest, put the book down, and resume the next day.

Remember, many people will find that, because of the poor habits we pick up over the years, the efficiency of our breathing will have deteriorated, and, as such, it can take a few weeks to see a difference in your health and symptoms. This book will guide you through the all important first five to ten days where you'll learn a variety of breathing exercises, many of which, once you've mastered them, you'll use for the rest of your life.

Go easy on yourself. This isn't a competition so there's no need to be competitive – even with yourself. Don't worry about failing – you can't. If you find yourself struggling, simply stop and come back to it the next day. And don't worry about not being able to master all the exercises first time either – if there are one or two you find tricky, skip over them and try them again in a week's time – you'll almost certainly find them easier then.

Do what you can – anything you do is positive. Simply follow the exercises in your own time and look forward to a lifetime of efficient and happy breathing.

So, if you're ready, let's move straight on to the first section, which explains the various symptoms that can be caused by inefficient breathing patterns. Do any of them sound familiar?

2

Symptoms Caused by Inefficient Breathing

Cold Hands and Feet

Many of us have cold hands and feet and put it down to poor circulation. We would not connect it to the business of breathing in and out. The word 'circulation' refers to the blood going around the body in the arteries and veins while it transports the oxygen to the tissues. The blood contains oxygen, and the only way we get oxygen into the body is by breathing it in. We don't get oxygen from food or from water, or from anywhere else apart from the air we breathe in. It therefore makes sense that if our breathing is not quite right, then it is possible that there might be something wrong with our oxygen levels, which might affect the circulation of blood going around the body. The whole lot is connected, and if you are plagued by cold hands and feet, you might just have found the answer!

Pale Face and Skin

Some people look rosy cheeked and healthy. Others look pale and never seem to get that healthy look. You may think you are pale because it's part of your genetic make-up, and that some of your family have the same type of skin. However, if you have some of the other symptoms listed in this book, your breathing may be under performing, and a few slight adjustments could change the way you look. After all, it's all very well looking 'pale and interesting' but if you also have cold hands and feet, have panic attacks and have needed a lot of dental work, maybe you should consider your breathing.

Difficulty in Catching Your Breath or Difficulty in Taking a Deep Breath

Do you have difficulty catching your breath, or are you unable to take a deep breath? Both of these may seem small problems to other people, but if you find you stop doing things, such as exercising, because you know you may not be able to breathe part way through the activity, then it can be very limiting for you. When was the last time you really filled your lungs, or sang your heart out, or ran really fast with no worries? Can you go out with your friends and laugh and laugh and laugh? Can you walk up a steep hill and still be able to breathe at the top? Is it your legs that let you down, or your breathing? Or do you have to hold yourself back (or take medication), so that you can control your breathing? If you have the slightest problem, then this book should really help you. If you feel a bit worried already, just drop your shoulders, relax, and read on.

Asthma

If you have asthma you may be aware of your breathing when you can't breathe (ie when your airways are tightening or when you are having an asthma attack) but you may not have considered your breathing when you are just sat at home minding your own business. Now is the time to start taking notice of your breathing. Are you breathing through your nose or your mouth at the moment? Can you feel the air going up your nasal cavities, or is it going past your throat, and slightly drying out your mouth? Most people with asthma breathe through their mouth at least part of the time, if not the majority of the time. You may be aware that you often have a dry mouth and need to drink a lot to keep your mouth moist.

Just by breathing through your nose all the time, instead of just some of the time, you should be able to have more control over your breathing and therefore your asthma.

Panic Attacks

Panic attacks are horrid! They can take over your life and make you feel miserable. You may not be aware of your breathing during the normal course of events, but the moment you start feeling panicky, you may feel you cannot catch your breath, you may try to escape, (for example leaving the room, the lift, or the building), and you may be in a state of collapse. You can often feel as if you are going to die. But take heart, nobody has ever died from a panic attack. By learning the techniques in this book, you should have much better control of your panic attacks and feel you can start doing all those things you would like to do, but without the dread, the worry, and without the panic.

Just a little bit of advice as you read this book: If any of the exercises make your panic worse, simply skip it and move onto the next. You may need to do the exercises in a different order than appears in this book. Take your time while trying the exercises – remember this isn't a competition, it's about you progressing at your own pace. If just by reading one of the exercises you can feel your panic rising, then simply read the exercise, rather than do it.

Asthma and Panic Attacks

Do you ever wonder if you are having an asthma attack or a panic attack? Have you been diagnosed with asthma but sometimes find the inhaler doesn't work? 40% of people diagnosed with asthma also have panic attacks. Once you have a better understanding of your breathing, you should be able to distinguish between the two, and take the appropriate action.

Hyperventilation Attacks

Hyperventilation attacks are similar to panic attacks but aren't as well known. They can occur at any time and have all the physiological symptoms but without any of the feelings of panic associated with panic attacks. They are often under reported and under diagnosed but are just as horrid as panic attacks. If you have an undiagnosed problem with fainting, or just feeling awful for no reason, you may be experiencing hyperventilation attacks.

Allergies, Eczema, and Skin Conditions

When we breathe too much air day in and day out, our bodies produce too much histamine. And excess of histamine 'over react' to normal, everyday things, such as dust, animals, and foods. The symptoms can often be seen on the skin and flare-ups often happen at times of stress. We can get into a cycle of stress leading to an increased breathing rate which, in turn, leads to an increase in our symptoms. By controlling our breathing we can control our symptoms and see them dramatically decrease.

Slack Jawline

If you breathe through your nose you will automatically use the muscles in the lower half of your face, making it look toned. If you let your mouth hang open, these muscles are not used and become slack, which can result in a gormless expression. (In my ten years' experience of teaching people to change from mouth to nose breathing, I saw many clients six to twelve months after I'd first seen them, and found many were unrecognisable as their face shape had changed so much. They also reported that friends they hadn't seen for a while expressed surprise at their changed appearance, asking such questions as 'have you lost weight?' or 'have you had a face lift?')

You might not have examined your jawline before, but as an experiment, just put your hands or fingers on your jawline and feel the difference in muscle tone as you change from breathing through your mouth to breathing through your nose.

Protruding Teeth

If you breathe through your nose, the muscles around the lips, and the lips themselves become strong, and keep the teeth correctly positioned inside the mouth. If, as a child, you breathed through your mouth for many years, your teeth may have protruded forward and you may have needed the attentions of an orthodontist and worn braces across your teeth. Many of my mouth-breathing clients had either protruding teeth, or had worn braces as children. It's now becoming a regular thing for orthodontists referring their patients to be taught how to breathe through their noses correctly.

Elongated Face Shape

Mouth breathers tend to have an elongated face shape rather than a round face shape. This is due to the position of the tongue in the mouth. If you breathe through your nose, your tongue is pushed up to the roof of the mouth, which over the growing years of a child, encourages the top row of teeth at the side of the mouth to widen. This allows the front teeth to stay in position, and stay snug behind the lips. The lips will be strong, not flaccid, and will hold the front teeth in position, creating a round shaped face.

If the mouth is open, the tongue falls to its base. This exerts no pressure on the upper side teeth, which tend to allow them to stay in a narrow position. As the lips are not closed, they have no effect on the front teeth, and they tend to protrude forward. The result of mouth breathing during the childhood and teenage years is to allow the face to develop a narrow elongated shape.

Dental Cavities

Many of us have had dental fillings at one time or another, but in my experience, people who breathed through their mouth part of the time, or all of the time, had many more fillings than nose-breathers. I put this down to the fact that if you breathe through your nose, the nasal passages filter out dust, germs, pollutants, and anything else in air. Conversely, there is no filter system in the mouth, and everything is breathed in straight over the teeth. Common sense tells us this can't be good for the teeth.

Repeated Chest and Throat Infections

As we've just seen, the nose is designed to filter out dust, pollen, germs, pollutants and anything else in the air. The air should ideally arrive in your lungs clean and warm. If you breathe through your mouth, the air will be the same temperature as it is outside, which could be quite cold, which could irritate your lungs. The air will also be unfiltered and could contain germs that someone else has just breathed out. When I started breathing through my nose all the time I noticed a marked reduction in the amount of colds and chest infections that I got. I also noticed that when I was ill, I had far fewer symptoms and they never seemed as severe as before.

Nasal Voice, Whispering Voice, and Losing One's Voice

If you are unable to breathe through your nose, you may have developed a nasal voice. This is not easy for other people to listen to, and you may sound as if you have a cold most of the time. You may also sound as if your sinuses are full of mucus – not the most attractive of things! Another common problem of mouth breathing is having a breathy, thin, or weak voice, or one that is no more than a whisper. This may be due to you breathing cold unfiltered air over your vocal chords. The good news is that by learning to breathe through your nose, and learning The Talking Exercise in particular, you may be able to improve your condition. Losing one's voice on a regular basis could also be connected to the same thing.

Abnormal Breathing Patterns

Are you aware there is something wrong with your breathing? Perhaps you get breathless with no reason. Perhaps you have difficulty in catching your breath, or sometimes have to try to control your breathing, and are unsure what to do. You may have some of the other symptoms in this book but had not connected them to your breathing. Visits to your doctor and a variety of medical tests may show there is no problem, you may have been handed an inhaler 'to see if it helps'. You may be left in a bit of a no-man's land, neither ill, nor completely well. In my experience, people who are in this category are chronically over breathing and mouth breathing the majority of the time. With this book, you might just have found the solution to your problem.

Snoring

When we go to sleep at night we are doing less than during the day and, as such, we breathe less. However, some of us breathe more than in the daytime, and in fact, so much air is rushing in and out of our noses or mouths when we are asleep, that a loud noise is emitted, which can be heard by other people. This is what we call snoring. The majority of people who snore would consider this a night time problem and assume that their breathing is 'normal' during the day, however, in my experience, snoring is often linked to inefficient daytime breathing. If they improve their daytime breathing, their breathing improves at night to the point where there is no longer any snoring. By learning to breathe the correct amount day and night, by practicing the exercises in this book, your night times may start being quieter.

Sleep Apnoea

Sleep apnoea is another problem seen in people who breathe too much at night. Their breathing patterns become abnormal, with a lot of breath-holding and the taking of huge breaths. It can be disturbing to listen to someone with sleep apnoea, as you can wonder if they will ever take a breath again, as the main symptom is that they actually stop breathing altogether for long periods. People with condition often are unaware that their daytime breathing is inefficient and if they restore normal daytime patterns, then their sleep apnoea tends to become less of a problem.

Lung Damage

If you have emphysema, Bronchiectasis, C.O.P.D. (Chronic Obstructive Pulmonary Disease) or any other form of lung damage, you probably have problems breathing during the daytime and at night, especially when you exert yourself such as when exercising. The secret of good breathing for you is to pace yourself so you don't start breathing through your mouth. Once you are breathing through your mouth you will have no control over your breathing, and that's when problems occur, which often results in you reaching for your medication. Pace yourself as you read through this book, don't worry about achieving anything, just try the exercises, and pick the ones that give you more control over your breathing

Hypertension/High Blood Pressure

When we measure our blood pressure, we are measuring the pressure exerted by the walls of the blood vessels on the blood inside the blood vessels. The walls of the blood vessels are surrounded by 'smooth muscle'. Smooth muscle is a type of muscle found in the body that wraps itself around the 'tubes' in the body, such as the airways, the blood vessels, and the intestines. We cannot control this type of muscle by flexing them or building them up at a gym. Smooth muscle is controlled by the level of carbon dioxide in the body. The level of CO_2 is determined by our breathing. Normalising your breathing patterns can normalise your blood pressure.

I.B.S (Irritable Bowel Syndrome)

The intestines, stomach, and bowel are 'hollows' or 'tubes' in the body, and are surrounded by 'smooth muscle'. Smooth muscle is a type of muscle that wraps itself around the tubes and hollows. This type of muscle cannot be controlled by trips to gym, or by working out. Smooth muscle is controlled by the level of carbon dioxide in the body. If there is too little CO_2, the smooth muscle tightens around the intestines etc, but once the correct amount of CO_2 is in the body, the smooth muscle loosens its 'grip' and the intestines are able to work normally. The amount of CO_2 in the body is determined by your breathing. If you have been struggling with IBS, you may just have found a solution.

3

THE MORE AIR YOU BREATHE, THE LESS OXYGEN YOU GET

So now we know some of the symptoms, let's try some breathing exercises to start to put things right. If you are wondering how I know all this information, I trained as a Buteyko Practitioner in 2000, and I've worked as one for the last thirteen years. I've taught hundreds of people to rectify their breathing, and all the advice and tips in this book come directly from my experience of teaching them. The advice in all of this book is based on the Bohr Effect. This, discovered and named after the scientist, Christian Bohr, showed that by breathing MORE air (into our lungs) we get LESS oxygen into our bodily tissues and the converse is true that by breathing LESS air into our lungs we get MORE oxygen. This is the opposite of what most people believe. A Russian doctor, Konstantin Buteyko, 'rediscovered' this information when he was undertaking his medical training in his home country. Buteyko practitioners are people who teach breathing exercises, based on this principle, worldwide.

So relax, drop your shoulders, and read on.

4

WHAT IS NORMAL BREATHING?

Normal breathing for an adult at rest, is breathing between 4 and 6 litres of air per minute, gently, through the nose. There are three parts to taking a breath:

1) the breath in

2) the breath out

3) the gap when nothing happens

It is the gap which is in many ways the most important part - something that few people are aware of, and crucially, if you can put the gap back into your breathing when things are going wrong, then you will be able to recover your breathing and get back to normal. I will explain how to do this in the section called How to Put a Gap in Your Breathing.

Breathing should feel effortless. Other people shouldn't be able to see or hear us breathe. There's no need to take in huge breaths in through the mouth, or using you shoulders or upper chest to breathe, or consciously moving our bellies in and out. Breathing is all done by our diaphragms. The diaphragm is a membrane that separates the chest cavity, that contains the lungs and heart, from our abdomen that contains our liver, kidneys, stomach and the other organs. It is a strong membrane made of muscle and it keeps the chest cavity airtight. If we can get our breathing correct, the diaphragm should do all the work for us, making us quiet and efficient breathers.

So, to work out where you're breathing from at the moment, do the following:

1) Sit on a chair. It should be a dining room or kitchen style chair, one with a flat back which keeps your

spine straight. Not an easy chair or one that you sink into.

2) To locate your diaphragm you need to put the end of your thumb on the base of your sternum in the centre of your chest, and the end of your little finger (of the same hand) on your belly button. Flatten your hand into your tummy and leave it there.

3) Next, put the other hand, spayed out, on your upper chest. (This is below your throat, and where you would find a necklace.)

4) Sit upright, there's no need to stretch up unnecessarily at this point, and see if you can feel where you are breathing from. Can you feel whether it is your upper hand, and therefore your upper chest that is moving as you breathe, or is it your lower hand and therefore your diaphragm, or is it both?

If you can breathe through your nose at the moment, you should be able to feel your lower hand moving. Try opening your mouth, and take a breath. Could you feel that as you changed your breathing to mouth breathing, your upper chest began moving?

If you feel you have understood everything so far then we can move on to the next exercise. If you feel you would like a bit more practice discovering how you are breathing at the moment, go back to the beginning of this section and repeat it. It is important you understand where you are breathing from before moving on.

If you have been unable to do this exercise because you can't breathe through your nose at all, move to the section entitled How to Clear Your Nose so You Can Breathe Through It. Then come back to this section.

You should breathe with your diaphragm when you are walking, talking, going upstairs, sleeping, working, and even running. It should only be necessary to breathe using your upper chest in instances such as when you are sprinting to finish a race, running for a bus, running away from danger, trying to beat someone at a sport. You will notice all these things are very active! But you may find that in the past you have often breathed through your mouth when you are walking along a road, shopping, doing housework, talking, sleeping, sitting at a desk or computer, and all manner of things.

So, to breathe with your diaphragm you need to make sure you are breathing through your nose at all times, rather than opening your mouth, which starts to use the upper chest. If you think of your daily tasks as a marathon, I want you to try and complete all your day breathing through your nose, and only breathe through your mouth when you are 'sprinting to the finish' or similar.

It's all very easy for me to say 'breathe through your nose all the time' and 'breathe using your diaphragm rather than your upper chest,' especially as you may not be used to doing that, so just relax, and read the next few chapters which explain exactly what to do.

Let's not forget what Buteyko and Bohr taught us:
THE MORE AIR YOU BREATHE, THE LESS OXYGEN YOU GET.

I have put this in capitals as it is so very important. It is also probably be the exact opposite of what you have believed before reading this book. In fact, in the past, you may have been told to take a deep breath. Did you interpret this to mean take a 'big' breath and filled your lungs? Many people think that if they breathe in a large amount of air, then they will get a large amount of oxygen into their lungs and that it would benefit their health. This is wrong. In actual fact, the more you breathe, the less oxygen you will get to your tissues.

So it makes sense to breathe through your nose rather than your mouth as your nasal passages are smaller than your open mouth. If you have been a mouth breather before, and are learning to change to nose breathing all the time, the quantity of air you now breathe could be substantially less than before. Remember this is a good thing, as the less you breathe, the more oxygen you will get to your tissues. You, like many others, may feel as though you're not getting enough air. It is *just* a feeling. This feeling could last about 24 hours, and can feel quite weird, as your body it telling you, 'you are not breathing enough,' and yet you seem to be fine, and even might look a bit pinker in the cheeks, or feel warmer in your hands and feet. If you get any of these weird feelings, just give yourself a break of 24 hours before you do any more of the exercises in this book. After all, you have probably been breathing incorrectly for years, so don't be surprised if it takes more than a day to master one thing.

5

WHAT TO EXPECT: CLEARING REACTIONS

When you make any changes to your breathing, it is possible you may have some side effects, or unpleasant reactions. These are called 'clearing reactions' and, whilst they're nothing to worry about, they can include

- Excessive tiredness

- Headaches

- Stomach upsets

- Sore back and chest muscles

- Mild depression

- Insomnia

- Excessive mucus production

- For children, a change in their energy levels

If you have any of these reactions, just go easy on yourself. Don't do anymore exercises today, just give yourself 24 hours to recover. Just keep trying to breathe through your nose. If any symptom lasts longer than 36 hours, then it is nothing to do with your breathing.

6

NOSE BREATHING Vs MOUTH BREATHING

Breathing the nose is important because the alternative is breathing through your mouth. The problem with breathing through your mouth is that you have no control over the amount you're breathing in. In addition, the air that you breathe in will be too dry for your lungs. Breathing dry air will cause the lungs to dry out which causes them to produce more of the mucus needed to lubricate them. Excessive mucus is a problem for many with breathing problems.

Another problem with breathing through your mouth is that you'll breathe in dust, pollen, and germs, which will go straight into your lungs without being filtered. Breathing through your nose is preferable because your nasal passages contain both hair and mucus which filter out these unwanted particles. Just imagine: on a sunny day when the sun shines in through your windows you will see lots of small particles in the air – if you're breathing through your mouth you'll be breathing them straight into your lungs. Once your lungs receive these particles their natural reaction is to cough in order to expel them.

Your lungs also prefer air that is the same temperature as they are. If you breathe through your mouth, the air going into your lungs will be the same temperature as it is outside (think of how cold it gets in winter!) whereas if you breathe through your nose the air is warmed as it passes through your nasal passages.

So it makes sense to always breathe through your nose. After all, the nose's main job is to warm, filter, and moisten the air going to your lungs. So let it do its job.

7

SHOULD I BREATHE IN THROUGH MY NOSE AND OUT THROUGH MY MOUTH?

I'm often asked whether we should breathe in through our noses, and then out through our mouths. This kind of practice is often encouraged in disciplines such as yoga, pilates, and tai chi, as well as other exercise programmes. The problem is that we breathe approximately twenty thousand times a day, and remembering to breathe in through our noses and then out through our mouths every time would be impossible.

Another problem is that changing from nose to mouth breathing changes the pressure in the lungs which is not good for them.

Therefore the answer is no.

You should just breathe in and out through your nose all day and all night which can be achieved by keeping your mouth closed.

Think of the lungs as a pair of old fashioned bellows - the sort you'd use to encourage a fire. Those bellows will have one small nozzle at the end where all the air is sucked in and puffed out of. As long as there's no tear in the material, the pressure remains the same and the bellows will work efficiently. Now, imagine the same pair of bellows, only these have a small hole in the material. Now we have a pair of bellows with two holes, so when the bellows are used the air is expelled through not one hole, but two, thus reducing air pressure and the bellows' efficiency. (Usually they're so inefficient they're thrown away.) This is the same as breathing through your mouth and nose, and it's why you should be breathing through your nose the whole time.

8

HOW TO CLEAR YOUR NOSE SO YOU CAN BREATHE THROUGH IT

If you have been unable to breathe through your nose until now, here's a great exercise you can do. It is a simple exercise and can be done at any time, and should be done whenever your nose is blocked.

Here's what you do:

1. Breathe in and then out.

2. Close your mouth..

3. Pinch your nose with your thumb and first finger so that no air can go in or out

4. Nod your head up and down for a few seconds (keeping your mouth closed).

5. When you feel you would like to breathe...

6. Remove your hand and breathe gently through your nose.

You may need to repeat this a few times to fully clear your nose. Tell yourself to relax, and drop your shoulders if they have crept up.

The Nose Clearing Exercise may be done as many times as you need. You may not need to do it ever again, but it is always a good idea to practice it, so that you can use it in the future if you need to. So do it a few more times now, learn to relax whilst you are doing it, and congratulate yourself for following my instructions so successfully!

For some people the above exercise is just not strong enough, so if your nose is not as clear as you'd like it to be, or it didn't clear at all, here's a different exercise which should help.

1 Stand up.

2 Breathe in and then out.

3 Close your mouth.

4 Pinch your nose with your thumb and first finger, so no air can go in or out.

5 Start walking as quickly or slowly as you like (most people like to go quite quickly).

6 When you feel you would like to breathe...

7 Remove your hand and breathe gently through your nose.

8 Sit down (and repeat if necessary).

Once you have mastered either of these exercises you can move on. If you feel you have already changed your breathing to a large extent, and feel like a rest, come back to this tomorrow.

For the next few days I'd like you to breathe through your nose at all times, using the nose clearing exercise whenever you need to. Practice keeping your mouth closed whenever you can, be it whilst walking around your house, or down the street, or down the corridors at work. Become aware of the situations where your mouth is open, and when you breathe through it and when you notice it is open, simply close it. Many of these situations, such as talking, sleeping, coughing, are covered later in this book. Watch out for breathing through your mouth when

- You have a pen in your mouth

- You look up

- You are amazed (at someone's amazing story!)

- Are looking in shop windows

- Are listening to someone

- Are watching TV

- Are reading

9

DO YOU NEED THAT NASAL SURGERY?

Are you contemplating nasal surgery to unblock your nose? This usually involves stripping out the lining of your nasal passages. I have taught people who were due to have this done, as well as people who had had it done in the past. The past patients had started with a blocked nose which they couldn't breathe through at all. Although the 'stripping out' surgery seemed to work initially, it didn't last for long and often the surgery had to be repeated. If you are contemplating having this surgery, I suggest you do two things. Firstly I recommend you unblock your nose using the nose clearing exercise you have already learned. You may need to do this a few times, maybe up to ten times in five minutes, to get your nose clear. The second part, which is the most important, is to keep your nose clear. It is likely to start blocking up again as soon as you start breathing through your mouth, so I recommend you learn all the exercises in this book.

10

HOW TO BREATHE IN AND OUT

Sounds simple doesn't it? But in my experience if you say to someone, 'breathe in and out' they take a large breath in through their nose or mouth, then breathe all the air out again. Remember: the more you breathe, the less oxygen you will get. I am never going to ask you to take a 'large' breath in. I don't want you to be breathing great big breaths.

Let's try now. Just sit where you are and let the air in through your nose and then let it out again. Try again and make sure you are just breathing a normal amount of air, not an increased amount.

This little exercise is important because many of the breathing exercises in this book begin with a breath in and a breath out, and those breaths should be small ones.

YOU SHOULD NOT BE ABLE TO SEE OR HEAR ANYONE BREATHING.

If you think of someone who is ill, perhaps with a respiratory illness, then their breathing will be loud and you'll be able to see their chest rising and falling. You may have noticed people in the past who've had terrible breathing. A healthy person should breath quietly and you should not be able to see their chest rising while they're at rest because they will be breathing the correct amount so there's nothing abnormal to see or hear, but you breathing might contain lots of sighs, sniffs, coughs or may just be noisy. If you follow this book your breathing should be noticeably quieter in a few days' time.

11

HOW TO PUT A GAP IN YOUR BREATHING

This exercise is possibly the most important of the whole book as it restores the breathing patterns to normal. It's one that can be used in a variety of situations. It's a simple exercise and possibly the one you will use the most often. What's more - it's effective even if you do it badly. And what is it? It's simply learning how to put a gap between your breaths, and it will stop your breathing running away with you. If you're ever unsure of which breathing exercise you need to do, simply go straight into this one.

As I mentioned earlier, normal breathing consists of three parts:

The breath in

The breath out

The gap when nothing happens

So let's just see what your breathing is doing at the moment.

Are there three parts to it:

IN

OUT

GAP

or, are there only two parts to it:

IN

OUT

If it is the latter then I would describe this as having no pause

(or gap) in your breathing.

There will be many times when you may be breathing without pause (i.e. no gap) and doing this exercise will be of benefit:

- When you are exercising. (By exercise I don't simply mean the vigorous kind you might do at the gym. It can also include walking and tackling the stairs.) It is normal for your breathing to increase and to have no gap when you are exercising.
- When you have finished exercising and are out of breath or recovering your breathing.
- If you are worried about something, or feeling apprehensive.
- If you are having a panic attack.
- If you are having an asthma attack.
- If you wake up with asthma symptoms.
- If you are breathing too fast, or too deeply.
- If you are feeling anxious or claustrophobic.

- If you are excited about something but you're not moving – even if that's only watching the TV.

- If your breathing is erratic.

- If you feel tight across the chest.

- If you feel a bit strange or feel you might faint.

- If you can't get to sleep.

There may also be times when you are just sitting reading the paper, or watching T.V. and you become aware that your breathing is not correct, or is running away with you. The feeling of your breath 'running away with you' is a common one, and is caused by not having that gap in your breathing. It feels as if you have no control of your breathing, and can be quite frightening, especially if you were just sitting there, minding your own business, and not doing anything exciting or unusual at the time.

Here's the exercise to put the gap back in:

(NB As you should be relaxed when you first practise this, the breaths in and out should be calm and normal. However, when you're doing this to normalise your breathing (ie trying to combat anything from the list above) do not worry about the sizes of the breaths. They are irrelevant. Just concentrate on putting the gap back in.)

- First close your mouth and let the air go in and out through your nose.

- At the end of the 'out' breath, pause and count to 2.

- Breathe in and out (twice if you need to).

- Pause and count to 2.

- Breathe in and out again (twice if you need to).

- Pause, and this time count to 3.

- Breathe in and out again (twice if you need to).

- Pause and count to 3.

- Breathe in and out again (twice if you need to).

- Pause, and now count to 2.

As you should be trying this exercise while your breathing is normal it shouldn't be too difficult. In fact this exercise is very easy to do, but you need to practice whilst your breathing is okay so that when your breathing is abnormal, or out of control, you can start this exercise and quickly regain control. Don't worry about the size or the breaths 'in' and 'out'. Just concentrate on putting the gap back in. Have another try at it now.

Don't worry about how long it takes to count up to two or three. When your breathing is bad, the '1, 2, 3,' may be very quick. But once you have been doing it for, let's say, one minute, you will you can space out the '1, 2, 3,' and your breathing will start to feel more under control.

Now I'd like you to have another try, and this time go up to four or five if you can, then come back down again to two.

During this exercise you can tell yourself to relax and drop your shoulders if they've crept up.

If you are getting the hang of it, read on. If you want some more practice, then go back to the beginning of this section and try the exercise again.

You can practice this as often as you like as it restores normal breathing patterns. If you are using the exercise to control your breathing in a certain situation you may do this exercise 20, 50 – or even 100 times – it doesn't matter, because it's all designed to get your breathing back to normal.

Further information:

- When your breathing pattern restores to normal, you will probably forget all about the exercise, and start concentrating on something else.

- If you want to, you can stay on the numbers 1, 2, and 1, 2, 3. There is no need to go higher if you don't want to. If you have lung damage, this will probably suit you best.

- Go up to number 6 if you are having a panic attack, there is no need to go higher.

- Go up to 10 if you are having an asthma attack.

- Don't push yourself to get higher numbers. If you are the competitive type, give up now! No one is going to reward you for getting to number 10! Just relax, and let the exercise bring your breathing back to normal.

- You can keep doing this exercise until you feel okay for example, before an interview, or if you feel trapped, or are feeling panicky. Just keep doing the exercise, up and down the numbers, in a non-competitive way.

12

HOW TO BREATHE THROUGH YOUR NOSE WHILST ASLEEP

An easy training aid, for day and night.

During the day it's easy to work out if you are breathing through your nose or your mouth. However, when you are asleep, you have no idea and consequently you have no control over your breathing. Breathing through your nose while you are asleep is an important thing to learn.

There are two ways of doing this. The first way is to employ somebody to stand watch over you all night and wake you up every time your mouth falls open (which I won't recommend as it is expensive and not practical!). A much easier, and cheaper way, is to place a small piece of micropore tape over your lips to keep them together. Micropore tape (readily available from chemists) is often used for holding bandages in place so it's perfectly safe to apply directly to the skin. It comes in a range of widths. For this, I'd recommend the narrowest width.

As the thought of taping your lips at night might make you feel uncomfortable I suggest having a practice during the day so you see that there's absolutely nothing to worry about.

Here's what I'd like you to do.

First, I'd like you to rip a thumb-sized piece off the role of tape. Next, we need to prepare it for use on your lips so I'd like you to stick it to your clothes (any are fine). Now, remove it and repeat the process. This funny little action removes much of the stickiness, and makes using it on your lips easier.

Next, sit somewhere relaxing and breathe through your nose for a little while. Make sure you are relaxed, and just put your finger (no tape yet) over your lips, as if telling someone to be quiet. Sit like this for a little while, and tell yourself 'I am sitting breathing through my nose, with my lips held together with my finger.' Next, remove your finger and place the tape over your lips and tell yourself: 'I am sitting breathing through my nose with tape holding my lips together.' Don't feel you have to completely seal your mouth. You should still be able to talk when the tape is on, even if it is through pinched lips. Sit like this for around half an hour. If you like you could put on the TV or some music, or maybe read a book (maybe even this one!).

It's possible that when you first try this you feel a little panicky – many people do. It's nothing to worry about and is a perfectly natural reaction. If this happens feel free to remove the tape, drop your shoulders, and relax and try again in a few minutes. If this exercise is still panicking you, just sit with your finger over your lips for a while. You may find that your arm is getting tired! It could be easier with a bit of tape! Try the tape again, and get used to it.

Okay, let's try this at night...

When you go to bed, just before you are about to go to sleep, lie down on your left side. If, at this point, your nose is blocked, you may need to clear it a few times before you're able to lie down. Relax, drop your shoulders. If you can't lie on your left, for some reason, lie on your right. And if you can't lie on either side lie on your front, but do not lie on your back. If you lie on your back, your mouth will naturally open and you will be breathing through it. If you lie on your side, in the foetal position, however, you will naturally breathe less as your lungs are squashed by your body position, and are therefore smaller, meaning you will breathe less.

Incidentally, if you have been standing up or sitting upright up for most of the day and then lie down, there is a lot of movement of blood around the body, and you may feel a bit breathless, uncomfortable, or even panicky. So just lie there until everything feels okay.

Now I'd like you to put your finger across your mouth as in the daytime exercise, then once you feel okay, put a piece of tape across your mouth. Don't panic. Remember, you can take the tape off at any time - no one is trying to suffocate you! Now, see if you can fall asleep with the tape on.

In my experience, one the following will happen:

- The tape comes off in the night and you'll find it on your bedclothes next morning.

- The tape is still over your lips in the morning.

- The tape is flapping around and only attached on one end.

- You pulled the tape off before you fell asleep.

- You pulled the tape off in the night.

- You find the tape days later!

The aim is to put the tape on each night and fall asleep whilst wearing it. You will have no control over it in the night. Do not worry about it. In many ways it is the easiest of all the exercises in this book as you sleep all the way through it!

What you will probably find, is that over the following few days and weeks, the tape stays on longer and longer. Remember, the aim of the tape is to keep you breathing through your nose all night. Do not put large pieces of tape over your mouth. After all, you are not a hostage! Do not use other forms of tape, and don't feel you have to completely seal your mouth. You should still be able to talk when the tape is on, even if it is through pinched lips.

Sweet dreams!

13

HOW TO SEND YOURSELF TO SLEEP WITH A BREATHING EXERCISE

Many of us have problems sleeping, whether it be nodding off when we first go to bed, or whether it's trying to return to sleep after waking in the night. This breathing exercise can help at both of those times. It's the same exercise as How To Put a Gap in Your Breathing. It's a lovely exercise for getting you off to sleep. You should only need to do it a few times and then, the next thing you know, it'll be morning. To save you flicking back through the book, here it is again:

- First close your mouth and let the air go in and out through your nose

   (If you struggle to breathe through your nose then you should complete the Nose Clearing Exercise first.)

- At the end of the 'out' breath, pause and count to 2.

- Breathe in and out (twice if you need to).

- Pause, and this time count to 3.

- Breathe in and out again (twice if you need to).

- Pause and count to 4.

- Breathe in and out again (twice if you need to).

- Pause, and now count to 5.

Keep going up through the numbers – all the way to 10, and you should find you fall asleep quickly and easily.

Good night!

14

HOW TO TAKE YOUR PULSE

If you want to monitor your condition in the future, I suggest you learn how to take your pulse. As you become accurate with it, try taking your pulse before and after some of the exercises in this book.

Here's how to do it. You will need a watch or clock with a second hand, and a pen or pencil and paper. I suggest removing your watch, if you wear one, and putting it on the table in front of you. Some people find it easier using a kitchen timer. (Some medications, including asthma medications, can make the ends of the fingers a bit numb, so this might hinder you in this exercise. If this is the case ask someone else to take your pulse for you.)

- Put your left hand on a table in front of you, palm up.

- Look at the tips of your fingers of your other hand - the parts that a policeman would use to take your fingerprints. Can you see that the 'fingerprint' areas are larger than the tips? As these parts of our fingers have a larger surface area, these are what we'll use to take our pulse, instead of the tips.

- Using all four fingers, on your right hand, run your fingers down the outside of the thumb of your left hand, until all four fingers are on the wrist.

- Creep your fingers in a little towards the centre of the wrist – roughly half way between the outside of your wrist and its centre.

- You should be able to feel your pulse under your skin here.

- Get used to the beat of your pulse. Relax and simply feel the beat for a few moments.

- Next, look at your watch or clock. Count the number of beats you feel from your pulse over a period of 15 seconds.

- Write that figure down. Multiply your number by four and you'll get your pulse rate per minute.

- Try this a few more times for practice. (Be careful you're not counting the seconds instead of your pulse by mistake.)

- I'd like you to repeat this a few times to improve your accuracy – it'll take a while to get used to it.

My clients are always asking me what a normal pulse rate should be. Well, the answer is very complex as there are so many things that can affect it: your age, your sex, how fit you are, medication, and what health problems you have. Your pulse rate will increase and decrease throughout the day, as you do different things. Your pulse will go up if you climb the stairs, listen to a thrilling play on the radio, drive a car at breakneck speed, play sports, eat food, etc. Your pulse will come down if you sit quietly reading a book, relax watching the T.V., listen to calming music etc. What's important is being able to take your pulse accurately so you'll be able to monitor it.

15

HOW TO MEASURE YOUR BREATHING: THE CONTROL PAUSE

If the last exercise was a way of measuring your pulse, this exercise is a way of measuring your breathing rate. You can do it anywhere - at home, at work, in the car, on your own and without needing anyone else's help. Having completed the Taking Your Pulse exercise you'll know that it took a few attempts before you'd mastered it. Well, the same thing applies here. In fact this will most likely take a few days for you to have mastered it completely.

Like the previous exercise, you will need a watch with a second hand, and a pen and a piece of paper.

- I'd like you to start by sitting down. Rest there for a few moments.

- Breathe in and out through your nose (remember, not huge breaths).

- Hold your nose closed with your finger and thumb (like you did for the nose clearing exercise).

- Count the seconds until you feel you want to breathe.

- When you want to breathe, release your nose and breathe normally through it.

- Write down the number of seconds.

Once you've read the next section I'd like you to try this exercise again.

Now I'd like to explain to you the processes involved in the exercise. The first instruction is to sit and have a little rest. Always do this when you are practicing because if you rush in, sit down and take your control pause quickly, the length of time will be very short. That's fine if you are measuring your breathing after physical exercise, but it doesn't help when you are learning.

The strangest part is the waiting, as the seconds tick by. You are waiting for your body to indicate when it needs to breathe. Your body might not tell you very much at this stage but don't be disheartened. This exercise, just like the pulse exercise, will most likely take about four or five days of regular practice to get right. In the early days, if you feel it isn't going as well as you'd like, relax, drop your shoulders, and don't panic. Remember: you *are* learning and this is probably the most difficult exercise to master.

Now let's check the 'breathe in and out' part. Remember not to take a huge breath in. This should mean you are only able to breathe the same amount out. Another thing to watch…

when you breathe out don't breathe all the air out of your lungs. When we breathe, two thirds of all the air in the lungs is inhaled and exhaled. One third stays in the lungs. The third that stays is actually in our airways. Don't worry, it's not at the bottom of your lungs going mouldy! As all the air gets mixed up, and is moving either in or out, there's no need to try to breathe all of it out. It is moving the oxygen in and the carbon dioxide out. It works perfectly well without you needing to think about it.

Does this exercise make you panic?

If you have panic attacks you may find this exercise makes you feel worse and brings on the feelings of panic. If that is happening to you, then simply stop doing it. Relax and drop your shoulders. It's time for you to have a break, so get up and have a walk around the room and, when you're ready, we can move on to the next section. You can always come back to this exercise in a few days' time – don't feel a failure - remember you *are* learning.

For those of you who do not have feelings of panic, I'd like you to try the exercise again and return here once you've done it.

The trickiest parts of the Control Pause are the beginning and the end. The bit in the middle whilst you are just sitting there holding your breath should be quite boring! So to repeat… the beginning should be:

- Breathe in
- Breathe out
- Hold your breath

The ending is a little different as it can take a few days before you perfect the art of knowing when your body wants to breathe again. There should be very little recovery needed from this exercise. Just one small breath, in and out. Certainly no large breaths, no opening of the mouth, no gasping. Having had a few tries at it, your endings may be all different. That's because you are a beginner!

You may be surprised to know that if you breathed the correct amount, that is between four and six litres of air per minute at rest, you would have a control pause of between 45 and 60 seconds.

At the moment, just try to be accurate. Remember, it is a measuring exercise, doing it lots of times will not make you better. And if you cheat, and hold your breath for longer than your body is telling you, you will have an inaccurate reading, which is of no use to anyone. Do this exercise four or five a day to practice. We will be using the Control Pause and pulse to monitor your breathing exercises further on in the book.

16

HORSE RIDER POSITION

This easy exercise is designed to reduce your breathing rate. Before we begin I'd like you to take your pulse. Then I'd like you to measure your Control Pause. We'll check them both again after the exercise to measure the effects, so be sure to write them down.

If you have been practicing the Control Pause and taking your pulse, as I suggested earlier, you should be more accurate than the first time you did them. So do them now, and remember not to artificially extend the control pause, after all, there is no reason to cheat!

The Exercise

This is not, for once, a breathing exercise, but instead a postural one that will have an effect on your breathing. For it you will need a clock, or watch, with a second hand - a kitchen timer or smartphone would do.

First I'd like you to sit on a straight-backed chair, such as a kitchen chair or dining room chair. Creep your buttocks forward until you are just sitting on the chair's edge. Let your arms dangle by your sides, or rest them, gently, palms up, on your thighs (as though you're about to be given a large bowl to hold), keeping your feet flat on the ground. DO NOT sit with your hands on your knees, with your arms straight and elbows locked, making your shoulders rigid and high. Bring your feet as far back under the chair as you can, without lifting any part of them off the floor. Keep them flat on the floor. If your feet don't touch the floor, (because you have short legs, or you are a child), put a cushion, stool or a thick book under your feet, or find a lower chair.

Now, 'lengthen your diaphragm' by stretching your body upwards, as though someone was pulling you up by a strand of your hair, leaving your arms where they were. You should feel 'perched' on the end of the chair. Although you should feel secure, if you leant backwards or forwards you would feel unstable and a bit wobbly. Sit there for two minutes. Let your shoulders drop. You are now in Horse Rider Position.

After two minutes, sit back in the chair, keeping your mouth shut. Just have a little rest. If you don't feel you can do two whole minutes, one minute or thirty seconds is fine.

Rest for two minutes.

If you feel okay, sit forward again into Horse Rider Position for another minute.

Then sit back and relax. Keep your mouth shut, don't talk, don't stretch, and keep your arms by your sides.

After two minutes, retake your pulse and Control Pause.

I'm sure you are analysing your results now! Your pulse should have either stayed the same or gone down. Your Control Pause should have gone up.

This is a gentle exercise and, depending on the overall state of your breathing, one of four things will have happened.

1) A total of 2 minutes was too much for you. Maybe your back ached, or you simply couldn't sustain the position for the full 2 minutes. If you come into this category, reduce the length of time you do this exercise for, say to 30 seconds each time, then gradually increase it. Don't worry too much about your pulse and Control

Pause readings at this stage. Practice them and write them down if you can.

2) Your Control Pause reading went up. Good. This amount of exercise, ie 3 minutes, is exactly correct for you.

3) This seemed to do nothing for you, and your pulse and Control Pause stayed the same. If this is the case, this exercise is too easy for you, increase the length of time you sit in the Horse Rider Position to three minutes each time, making six minutes in total.

4) Although the Horse Rider position went well, the pulse and Control Pause went wrong! Do not worry. You are still a beginner and still learning.

- If your back hurts whilst you do the Horse Rider Position then just sit back, you have done enough for the time being.

17

A DAILY PLAN FOR A BEGINNER

By now you should be familiar enough with the exercises we've covered so far that we can incorporate them into a daily plan. I'd like you to do a SET of exercises...

A SET of exercises consists of

1. Taking your Control Pause and writing it down.

2. Taking your pulse and writing it down.

3. Checking there is a gap in your breathing.

4. Sitting in Horse Rider Position (see previous chapter for your starting time, ie are you starting on 30 seconds, one minute, two minutes or three minutes) – writing down the length of time you sat for.

5. A 2 minute rest

6. Sitting in Horse Rider Position again (30 seconds, 1 min, 2 mins or 3 mins).

7. Another 2 minute rest.

8. Taking your control pause and writing it down.

9. Taking your pulse and writing it down.

Day One

Do one set of exercises before breakfast.

Do one set of exercises before lunch.

Do one set of exercises before bedtime.

Day Two

Increase the length of time you do the Horse Rider Position.

Increase it by one minute. If you feel you want to go slower, and repeat Day One, then that's fine. It is not a race.

Do one set before breakfast.

Do one set before lunch.

Do one set before evening meal.

Do one set before bedtime.

Days Three, Four and Five

Increase the length of time you do the Horse Rider Position. Increase it by one minute, up to a maximum of five minutes. Do five or six sets of exercises today

From Day Six Onwards

Do six sets of exercises a day, for up to five minutes each horse rider position session. This means each set will consist of ten minutes, and if you do six sets, this will mean you sit in horse rider position for a total of sixty minutes a day.

If you have got a bit lost with all the sets, just go back to the beginning, and take each day as it comes.

After the first week, you should have a good idea what you are doing. You may decide not to keep taking your pulse and control pause, but simply do the Horse Rider Position. This is fine, after all, it is the Horse Rider Position that will help change your breathing, the pulse and control pause are just monitoring its effects. However, in my experience, people who never write anything down, can forget to do the exercises, and never make much progress. So get into the habit of doing your first set of exercises first thing in the morning, writing it all down if you can. This way you can monitor what is happening to your breathing, and it will serve as a reminder to do it as well.

18

DON'T SRETCH!

You may be wondering why I am telling you not to stretch.

Well, consider this: Think about how big your lungs are.

They fill up the space in your chest cavity, along with your

heart. If you keep your arms by your sides and curl up in the

foetal position, (you can try this sitting on a chair, you don't

have to lie on the floor) you will physically be squashing

your lungs and they will therefore only be able to expand a

relatively small amount. Now sit up, stretch your arms above

your head (as if you are being held at gunpoint). Can you tell

that you have increased the physical size of your lungs? They

are quite a bit larger now that you have opened up your chest

cavity. It is possible for you to breathe large amounts of air,

but remember, the more you breathe, the less oxygen you

will get.

Now relax again, and put your arms by your sides. Your lungs will be able to breathe less air. Now, I don't want you to do this exercise again, but I want you to remember it. As you change your breathing, and breathe less day by day, your body may react by deciding to have a good old stretch! As soon as you are aware you are about to stretch, bring your arms down by your sides, and congratulate yourself for remembering such a peculiar instruction!

19

IS IT POSSIBLE TO BREATHE THROUGH YOUR NOSE WHILST YOUR MOUTH IS OPEN?

If you try this now you will discover it is entirely possible, and quite easy too (just think to how you have to breathe when you're in the dentist's chair). But to enable us to do it, we have to concentrate, as it feels like we have to 'shut off' part of the back of the throat. As soon as we stop concentrating, we will just revert to breathing through an open mouth. So as a general rule, if your mouth is open, and you're not thinking about it, you will be breathing through it.

RELAX AND DROP YOUR SHOULDERS

As you already know, tensing up and raising your shoulders is a common reaction to anyone learning new breathing exercises. The problem is, when this happens, it hinders the body's ability to breathe solely with the diaphragm, as raised shoulders increases the space in the lungs resulting in you being able to breathe more air than you need. (Remember, the more you breathe, the less oxygen you get.) So, as you try the different breathing exercises, try and remember to drop your shoulders as they may have a tendency to creep up round your ears. If you are perfectly relaxed at the time, and your shoulders are relaxed, just skip over this instruction and move on to the next thing.

HOW TO STOP COUGHING

There are a number of reasons why we cough. The first is because we've inhaled an unwanted particle, such as dust, which the lungs immediately reject. The second is when a particle of dust is lodged in the lungs. The lungs will produce mucus which surrounds the particle. This irritates the lungs and so we will cough that up too.

If you have a cold or flu-like illness, the lungs may well be irritated and inflamed, in which case they will produce mucus to lubricate the airways. In this case there will be more mucus in the lungs, and, eventually, that will be rejected as well.

In these above three cases, if the cough produces mucus, there is no need to worry.

If, however, you have a dry or tickly, unproductive cough (ie one which does not produce any mucus) repeated coughing can damage the lungs. Often this type of cough leads to a coughing spasm or lack of control over the cough, which can be painful.

Some facts about coughing

- A soft cough, a little like a false cough an actor might do on stage, will assist mucus to move. But a large cough will damage your airways.
- You might find you cough more as you start to change your breathing. Don't worry, you are probably clearing old mucus out of the lungs.

To avoid damaging the lungs, as soon as you feel you are about to cough, do one of the following. They may take practice.

- If you need to cough, cough with your mouth shut. As soon as you cough (which is a breathing-out action) close your mouth and breathe in through your nose. This means that the next breath of air going into your lungs is warmed, filtered and moistened - just what your lungs want. If you breathe through your mouth by mistake you will be breathing in cold, dry, unfiltered air, which will irritate your lungs, meaning more mucus and more coughing later. So clamp that mouth shut!

- How to stop a cough in the first place. When you feel you are about to cough take in three quick sniffs, all through your nose. Next, pause. Hold your breath until you want to comfortably breathe again. When you're ready, gently breathe out through your nose. (Incidentally, this is the only exercise in the whole book where I'll ask you to hold your breath once you've breathed in, ie with the lungs inflated.

Something else you could try when you feel you're about to cough is this exercise:

Breathe all the air out of your lungs slowly - including that third that normally stays in the airways. 'Hold' for a little while, (this means 'wait,' similar to waiting during the Control Pause), and then slowly breathe in again through the nose.

The last three exercises will need practice, so I'd suggest trying them now. Just remember to not ever make yourself cough as it is very damaging to the lungs.

Two other ways of stopping coughing are:

- Suck a boiled sweet. A medicated lozenge is not necessary as it is the sucking action that is thought to calm the coughing reflex.

- Have a sip of water, warm if possible.

Tickly cough. Or wanting to cough up mucus from deep within the lungs.

Do you sometimes feel as if you have a bit of mucus at the base of your lungs and you think the only way to get it out is to cough it up? We all know how that feels – it's as though only a huge cough will shift the mucus. It often takes numerous big coughs to dislodge a small amount of mucus. This is very damaging to the lungs.

I have an alternative for you: just let the bit of mucus reabsorb into your lung tissue. So, instead of bracing yourself and producing a lot of effort to do some big coughs, sit back and relax. Although the 'irritating' feeling stays for a while, you will find you can put up with it. You will discover that nothing bad happens, and you can relax a bit longer. If your lungs really want to get rid of that bit of mucus they will cough it up, so don't worry about that.

22

HOW TO STOP SNEEZING

Sneezes often come from nowhere and can surprise us, in which case there's not much you can do to stop them. But sometimes we can feel we are about to sneeze, and it can feel as if the whole world stops. You may tell someone else, 'I'm going to sneeze,' as if it's the most important thing they are going to hear that day! Of course they are not really all that interested, but they will often stop everything they are doing just to wait for your sneeze! It is during this time you can try a little action that may just stop it.

Here's what you should do. Place your forefinger above your top lip as though you are doing an impression of someone with a moustache. Now, with that finger, push back as though you were trying to push your head backwards. This funny little action, as well as often stopping an imminent sneeze, can also be used if you start sneezing and are unable

stop.

HOW TO STOP YAWNING

Yawn with your mouth closed. If you do yawn, pretend someone important like Her Majesty the Queen is stood next to you. You would try and stifle a yawn then wouldn't you? So try to keep your lips together. You will end up pulling a funny face, but at least it'll have stopped you yawning. Try to make sure the air goes in and out of your nose rather than your mouth.

24

HOW TO STOP SIGHING

Actually, it's very difficult to stop sighing (which you're probably doing now after reading this!). Try to be aware if you sigh a lot. Just try to control your breathing as best you can. As you change your breathing your body might try to 'sneak in' a bigger breath by sighing. Try to stop these sighs as soon as they start.

HOW TO STOP HICCUPS

Hiccups can be funny at first, but annoying if they persist. But they CAN be stopped! Here's how...

You may remember this from the coughing section!

Slowly breathe out all the air in your lungs (including the third that normally stays in the airways.) Wait for a few moments until you feel you want to breathe again. Then when you do, you should slowly breathe in again through your nose. You may need to repeat this a few times. Often the hiccups disrupt this exercise, so just persevere, repeating the exercise until they stop. It is best to practice this exercise a few times so you can use it whenever you need to.

A DAILY PLAN FOR AN INTERMEDIATE

Now that you've mastered the Daily Plan For Beginners, you're ready to move on to this, a Daily Plan for An Intermediate. This plan has the same format and timings as the Beginners' Plan, but this time you'll be adding a breathing exercise to The Horse Rider Position.

To begin with, you'll need a clock, a pen, and some paper. Now, let's get familiar with The Horse Rider Position again. Sit on a chair, perched at the end, feet flat on the floor (and back a bit), your body stretched up as if someone is pulling your hair up to the ceiling.

Once in this position, become aware of your breathing and, for about 30 seconds, reduce the amount you are breathing, so you are slightly under-breathing. Imagine you are playing hide and seek with someone. You decide to hide behind a full length curtain (perhaps in a doorway). Once behind the curtain, you will have to breathe very quietly, in fact slightly under-breathe, otherwise you will be heard and found. Imagine the seeker is standing on the other side of the curtain. Remember, they might stay there for a long time. This breathing is called 'reduced breathing' but you may want to remember it as 'behind the curtain' breathing.

So after 30 seconds of behind the curtain breathing, return to normal breathing.

Now give yourself a few minutes' rest, then you can try it again.

If you got a headache, felt faint, or dizzy, come back to this section another day. Don't be disheartened, relax and continue with the beginners' plan for a few days.

Assuming you are okay, have another go in a minute or so.

But before you do, read the following:

This exercise consists of slightly under-breathing for a few minutes. Later, we are going to do two minutes, so don't try and make it so hard that you can't sustain it. You should not feel you are restricting yourself, or strangling yourself. You will probably fluctuate between reducing your breathing and breathing normally. That's fine for the moment.

So have a go now.

Time yourself for one minute and, slowly, reduce the amount you are breathing, so you are just breathing a bit less than normal. If it feels awful, then you are reducing the volume far too much, so relax, and have another go.

Okay. So once the one minute is over, it will take up to 90 seconds for your breathing to recover. So sit back in your chair, relax, with your mouth closed.

Ask yourself how you feel. If you feel weird, ill, dizzy, sick, or have a headache, go back to the Beginners' Plan for a few days, and try again.

If you feel okay, after a little rest, I'd like you to try two minutes.

This time, I want you to take a Control Pause and take your pulse first, then do two minutes 'behind the curtain' breathing, then take your control pause and pulse again.

Have a go now, and write it all down. We write down reduced breathing as RB, so two minutes reduced breathing is written as 2min RB.

So here's the SET of exercises for the intermediate daily plan:

A SET of exercises consists of

1. Take your control pause and write it down.

2. Take your pulse and write it down.

3. Check there is a gap in your breathing.

4. Sit in Horse Rider Position and slowly reduce your breathing for 2 minutes.

5. Rest for 2 minutes.

6. Sit in Horse Rider Position again, reduce your breathing for 1 minute

7. Rest for 2 minutes.

8. Take your Control Pause and write it down.

9. Take your pulse and write it down.

Day One

Do one set of exercises before breakfast (2 minutes Reduced Breathing (RB), and then 1 minute as above).

Do one set of exercises before lunch (2min RB, then 1 min RB).

Do one set of exercises before bedtime (2 min RB, then 1 min RB).

Day Two

Increase the length of time you do the Horse Rider Position with Reduced Breathing. Increase it by one minute. If you feel you want to go slower, and repeat Day One, then that's fine. It is not a race.

Do one set before breakfast (3 mins RB, then 2 mins RB).

Do one set before lunch (as above).

Do one set before evening meal (as above).

Do one set before bedtime (as above).

Days Three, Four and Five

Increase the length of time you do the Horse Rider Position with Reduced Breathing. Up to a maximum of five minutes each RB session.

Do five or six sets of exercises today (5 mins RB, then 5 mins RB).

From Day Six Onwards

Do six sets of exercises a day, for up to five minutes each Horse Rider Position with Reduced Breathing session. This means each set will consist of ten minutes, and if you do six sets, this will mean you sit in horse rider position with reduced breathing for a total of sixty minutes a day.

27

STAND UP AND SIT DOWN AGAIN

Before we go any further I'd like you to stand up and sit

down again.

'What's the point of that?' I hear you ask. Well, try it and see

if you can notice what's happening with your breathing.

Did your mouth open when you got up? If you're like most

people it did. Now, try it again, this time make sure your

mouth stays closed when you get up and sit down.

Checking your mouth is closed when doing simple actions,

such as sitting down, is something you can easily incorporate

into your everyday routine. And it isn't only applicable to

getting up and sitting down. If you groan or moan when you

get up then your mouth is sure to be open. Now try a few

more activities, such as getting the vacuum out of the

cupboard, leaning down to pick something up off the carpet, leaning across a table, stretching up into a cupboard, getting into a hot bath, getting under the shower, doing the vacuuming, looking in a shop window, getting into the car, patting the dog, stroking the cat, putting on your socks. You can see there are hundreds of daily activities where your mouth could be opening without you noticing. If you have been putting what you've learned from this book into practice you may have noticed your mouth opening on some occasions. In fact, noticing when your mouth is open is the first sign that you are starting to change your breathing.

28

ARE YOU ALWAYS SMILING, OR ALWAYS TALKING?

Smiling, it is generally accepted, is a good thing. It shows that we're happy and studies have shown that simply seeing someone else smiling has a positive effect on our own well-being. And while, of course, I want you to be happy and would never suggest not smiling, I would ask you to keep in mind that when you do, your mouth tends to be open, and when our mouths are open we tend to breathe through them. And, as we already know, that leads to us taking in more air than we need, which means we're getting less oxygen than we need too. If you're happy, try to be happy while breathing through your nose.

If you are a chatterbox, and never stop talking, you may be breathing through your mouth all the time. Become aware of how you breathe whilst you talk and learn the Talking

Exercise which is coming up next.

29

HOW TO BREATHE THROUGH YOUR NOSE
WHILST TALKING

Many people breathe through their mouths when they speak. Are you one of them? Let's see.

Say, out loud: 'Hello, I live in a house.'

Did you notice whether you breathed through your mouth or your nose before you said 'Hello'?

Try this now:

- Breathe in through your nose.

- Open your mouth and breathe out as you say: 'Hello, I live in a house.'

- You may feel your chest collapsing a bit as you said that – which is perfectly normal at this stage.

- Close your mouth and breathe in again.

  Now, let's try that again. Make sure you speak out loud. You cannot do this exercise silently in your head!

- Breathe in through your nose.

- Breathe out as you say: 'One, two three, four.'

- Close your mouth, and wait until you want to breathe in again.

- Breathe in through your nose.

- Breathe out as you say: 'Five , six, seven.'

- Close your mouth, and wait again.

- Breathe in through your nose.

- Breathe out as you say 'eight, nine, ten.'

I'd like you to repeat that a few times so you get used to it. Once you are, I'd like you to replace the numbers with these short sentences.

- Breathe in through your nose as before.

- When you breathe out I'd like you to say: ' Hello I live in a house.'

- Make sure your mouth is closed, wait.

- Breathe in through your nose again.

- Breathe out as you say: 'It has a door and windows.'

- Close your mouth, wait.

- Breathe in through your nose.

- Breathe out as you say: 'We have pictures on the walls.'

Now I'd like you to practise using a few sentences of your own. Drop your shoulders and relax. When you first start talking like this it can feel as if you are speaking far too slowly, but, rest assured, people will find it easy to listen to. However, just like all the exercises, it takes practice, and it's often best to practice on your own.

If you find talking to yourself a bit peculiar, pretend you are showing someone round your house, and describe in detail the different pictures, chairs, ornaments, and anything else that you could talk about. Practice talking whilst standing up, and sitting down, but don't talk whilst you are walking. Talking in this way and walking at the same time can be tricky, and can be left for a few weeks, when you have mastered the basics.

There are three things that people often do that I'd like you to avoid.

1 Don't hold your breath when you speak. If you do this, you will have to breathe out a large breath at the end of your sentence. Let the air out *as* you speak.

2 As you speak, do not keep talking for a long time as you will run out of air, and feel as if your chest is collapsing. Stop after a few words, close your mouth, breathe in again through your nose, then speak again.

3 Don't breathe in a large breath, then only say a few words (ie, not enough) then breathe in again. You will start to inflate your lungs and feel as if you are going to burst! Just talk a few more words than you were before.

If you find that you are making some of the mistakes I've mentioned above, don't be disheartened, and don't give up. Tell yourself to relax again and go back to counting the numbers as shown in the first talking exercise.

Once you start breathing like this, you may notice the way other people breathe when they speak. Television presenters are interesting to watch, as some will breathe through their nose, and are easy to listen to. Others mouth-breathe and seem to be breathing all the air in the studio!

If you do any public speaking, or teaching large numbers, this exercise could improve your delivery. Once mastered, you will sound under control, not at all nervous, and will be easy to listen to and what you say will be clear. Your audience will be able to relax as they listen to you. If you have to answer a question, remember to breathe in through your nose before you answer. This also gives you a split second longer to prepare your answer, and gives you a controlled manner, which should impress your audience!

30

HOW TO BREATHE THROUGH YOUR NOSE
WHILST EXERCISING

Being able to breathe through your nose, rather than your mouth, whilst exercising will enable your body to work efficiently which, if you follow my instructions and practice, you can learn to do without becoming breathless. And that means you'll be able to comfortably exercise for longer, and more efficiently too. By breathing through your nose whilst you are 'moderately' exercising means you'll get a more efficient uptake of oxygen by your whole body.

NB When I mention exercise I mean all of its connotations – that can be anything from a gentle walk to a heavy gym session, or even something as demanding as a triathlon.

The key of nose-breathing whilst exercising is to start slowly.

When exercising, what I'd like you to aim for is to breathe

through your nose throughout the duration of the session,

only opening your mouth to breathe when you're pushing

yourself a little harder, such as sprinting to the finish, or

putting on an extra burst, maybe to climb to the top of a hill.

People fall into one of the following three categories:

1

Some people never exercise, and sometimes that's because

they always seem to end up breathless and feeling worse, not

better, after exerting themselves. If you fit into that category,

here's what I'd like you to do.

Start by standing up and before you set off, make sure you

are nose –breathing and that there is a gap in your breathing.

This may take a few minutes to achieve. Once you've achieved it, drop your shoulders, and walk slowly round your house, or your garden, or set out from your front door. As soon as you feel your breathing is speeding up, or that you want to open your mouth, stand still for a while and get your breathing back to normal. You may have only walked a few steps or be halfway down the road. It doesn't matter how far you have gone. When you have recovered, start walking slowly again, breathing through your nose, stopping as soon as you need to. Keep stopping and starting but do not allow your breathing to increase to the point you need to open your mouth to breathe. Once you have finished, whether you have been walking for two minutes or twenty, sit down, making sure you are still breathing through your nose. Then have a rest.

I suggest doing this a few times a day, each time controlling your breathing. After about a week you will probably find you can go further, or faster, whilst continuing to nose breathe. You can now consider yourself to be 'exercising' and can move on to the next section.

2

If you feel you can walk reasonably well, perhaps you often go out walking, then go to your venue as usual. Try and pick somewhere with no hills or inclines. Start by standing still and make sure you are breathing through your nose. Set off at a slow pace. In a relaxed manner, just walk along the track, path, or road, making sure you are breathing through your nose at all times. As soon as you feel that your breathing is getting too fast, or too deep, or you want to open your mouth, just stop. Get your breathing back to normal by putting a gap in your breathing. Relax and drop your shoulders. Do not worry about how far you go, or that you are walking slowly. As the weeks go on, you will get faster and be able to go for longer walks.

3

If you go cycling, running, or play team sports on a regular basis I suggest you spend approximately a week on number 2. Once you are walking fast, try breaking into a run, but make sure your mouth is still closed. Every time you feel your breathing is getting out of control, halt and recover your breathing. Then start again. Consider that if you were running a marathon, you would run the first 25 miles breathing through your nose and only mouth breathe as you sprint to the finish. It will probably be necessary to mouth breathe as you run up hills, or overtake a competitor, but as soon as you return to 'just' running, go back to nose-breathing. During team sports, there are times when you are very active, and will probably be mouth breathing, but the rest of the time, you should be nose-breathing. As you will have to concentrate on the game, you will probably forget about your breathing. The secret is to keep saying to yourself: 'Close your mouth, close your mouth, close your mouth!'

Use your nose as a gauge, if it starts to block, then you are going too fast. Although it can be quite annoying to go so slowly at the beginning for someone who is fit and active, within a week you should be back to your normal speed, but breathing through your nose all the time instead of breathing through your mouth. As you become a better breather, you will get more oxygen to your tissues, which should make you a better athlete.

31

FOOD AND BREATHING

We eat, on average, between three and six times a day, and every time we eat our breathing rate temporarily increases. Although eating any kind of food will increase our breathing rate, some foods increase it more than others. The two groups that do this the most are proteins and stimulants. The information in this section is not nutritional advice, nor is it a diet, nor a list of foods to avoid. However, if your breathing is poor at the moment (for example your Control Pause is less than 20), then you may get symptoms, such as breathlessness, tightness in the chest, panicky feelings, coughing, sneezing or raised shoulders after eating a particular food from the list. Simply knowing the following list should help you with controlling your breathing in the future. Also, note that the faster a food is digested, the faster it will increase the breathing rate.

If your Control Pause is low, and your pulse is high, then eating anything on the following list will increase your breathing rate, making your breathing effectively worse which may result in you having symptoms. However, if you master the exercises in the book and improve your breathing (getting your Control Pause higher than 30, 40, or higher) you should be able to eat them without any ill effects.

To test this out on yourself, take your Control Pause and pulse, eat a food you wish to test, and re-take your Control Pause and pause 20 minutes later.

Here's a list of foods that increase the breathing rate more than others. They are primarily proteins and stimulants.

- **Milk (this includes cows', goats', and soya, but does not include rice milk).** This is liquid protein and is absorbed quickly, resulting in an increased breathing rate within a short time.

- **Yogurt, soft cheese and ice cream** are milk based, easy to digest, and have a similar effect to milk. Harder cheeses take longer to digest and have a slower, almost non-existent effect.

- **Fish, tofu and chicken.** All are protein and are digested much faster than lamb, beef or pork.

- **Stock. Chicken, beef and fish stock** are liquid protein. Don't forget, stock is often an ingredient in sauces and gravies.

- **Honey.**

- **Nuts.**

- **Chocolate**, including drinking chocolate.

- **Berries**. All berries, such as strawberries and raspberries, contain chemicals called salicylates, which increase the breathing rate. (By the way, as I'm often asked... grapes are not berries so are not included.)

- **Alcohol.** A small amount of alcohol acts as a relaxant, but large amounts increase the breathing rate.

- **Caffeine.** This includes coffee, strong tea, cola drinks and some canned drinks.

32

WHAT TO DO IF YOU HAVE A COLD OR FLU

When you are ill your breathing rate increases because your body is under stress. What we need to do is to make sure that you don't inadvertently increase it further. All the same principles apply when you are ill, as when you are well. You may feel that you are far too ill to be doing any breathing exercises, but in fact you should be doing even more!

Here's What To Do

Always breathe through your nose. Once your mouth is open you will have lost control of your breathing, so use the Nose Clearing Exercise as often as you need to. You may find that you can sit on the sofa watching TV breathing through your nose, but as soon as you get up to do something, your nose blocks. This is your body telling you to sit down and rest!

Try and be guided by your nose. If, every time you do an activity, your nose blocks up, then stop doing it. By activities I mean walking upstairs, unloading the dishwasher, chatting on the phone, working, walking – it could be ANYTHING! The more you rest the better you will feel.

I recognise that in this day and age, resting at home is not considered the thing to do when one is ill. Television adverts suggest we should take some medication and carry on with our day as if nothing was wrong. However, from a breathing point of view, it is better to stay at home and rest when you are ill. However, there is no need to sleep more. Resting is just fine.

Do not oversleep. You may know from experience that, when you are ill, if you sleep for a long period, you can feel ghastly when you wake up. It can take all morning to recover. That is because sleeping for a long time is a huge stress on the body, and the breathing rate can increase as the hours go by. So see if you can wake yourself up after about four hours sleep, do some exercises from this book, and go back to sleep again.

Do not overeat. Remember that list of foods earlier in the book? This is a good time to avoid them all.

Drink lots of fluids, you will be sweating more, producing mucus, coughing more and could be getting dehydrated.

Don't do physical exercise as you will increase your breathing rate even more.

Do between six and nine sets of exercises each day, either from the beginners' plan or the intermediates'.

33

THE MINI PAUSE - THE BUTEYKO PRACTITIONER'S FAVOURITE EXERCISE!

I hope you are getting a good grip of your nose breathing, and are progressing and noticing the benefits in lots of different ways. This next exercise, called the Mini Pause, is such a funny little exercise you might wonder why anyone would tell you about it.

Here's what you do:

Breathe in and out (no large breaths remember, and don't empty your lungs).

Hold your breath for between 2 and 5 seconds.

Breathe normally again.

Yes, that's it! If you have struggled to understand and practice some of the other exercises, you may be wondering if you've missed a page of instructions! You haven't missed anything. The Mini Pause really is that simple! Now I'm going to tell you when you could use this.

After you have coughed, sneezed, yawned or sighed. Do you remember earlier I advised you how to stop doing these things? They all involve large breaths which is the opposite of what I'm advising you to do. So whether you are able to keep your mouth closed or not, do a Mini Pause after you have coughed, sneezed, yawned or sighed. It will help balance your breathing, and give you a little more control. Only one Mini Pause is required.

If you get a lot of nasal congestion before going to sleep. Do this exercise often in the fifteen minutes before you go to sleep - there's no limit on how many times you can do it.

You can do it sitting up in bed, or lying down. It's important to get your nose clear before you fall asleep, so you can breathe through your nose all night. It is also essential if you are putting the tape over your lips as mentioned earlier in the book.

If you have got a cold, or flu, then do one hundred Mini Pauses a day, each day that you are ill. Yes. One hundred! I suggest doing them in batches of ten, spread out through the day. Keep a record, by writing the number down, and keep the bit of paper in full view. It will remind you to do some more later! Doing one hundred Mini Pauses a day is thought to boost the immune system.

34

WHAT DOES MY CONTROL PAUSE READING MEAN?

By no you should have had lots of practice at the Control Pause, but you may be wondering what your readings mean. If you have normal breathing, you should have a Control Pause of between 45 and 60 seconds. This may seem very high to you at the moment, but if you have been keeping records and practicing the various breathing exercises, you may have noticed your Control Pause has gone up since Day One.

Remember the important things about the Control Pause.

• When you started you weren't very accurate, so some of your readings for the first few days may be far too high, very low, or just plain weird!

- Do not try to force your Control Pause higher than it is. Remember it is a measurement, just like taking your pulse.

- Doing lots of control pauses will not improve your health (just as taking your pulse will not make you better).

- If you breathing improves, your Control Pause will go up.

- If your breathing deteriorates, your Control Pause will go down.

- About 5% of people are never accurate with their Control Pause. If you are one of these people, don't worry about it. Use a different monitoring system for your health, such as your pulse, or how much medication you need to take.

When you do your Reduced Breathing Exercises, or Horse Rider Position (if you remain on that exercise) then your Control Pause should go up after the exercise. Wait for 90 seconds after your Reduced Breathing Exercise before taking your Control Pause.

Your Control Pause should go up after physical exercise as long as you have been breathing through your nose for the majority of the time. Wait a couple of minutes after exercise to regain your breath and recover slightly before measuring your Control Pause.

WHAT TO DO IF YOU HAVE AN ASTHMA ATTACK

The breathing exercise to do, if you can feel your airways tightening, is a Control Pause and then five minutes Reduced Breathing. Then, a second Control Pause, and another five minutes Reduced Breathing. If your condition is improving you can repeat the above sequence. But do not spend longer than 20 minutes trying to control your breathing with these exercises as you will get worn out. If, at any stage, you feel the breathing exercises are not helping, then take one puff of your reliever medication, wait for five minutes to let it work, then, if necessary, take another puff of your reliever medication. If you do not have your reliever medication to hand and you are unable to control your breathing you need to request emergency medical assistance.

WHAT TO DO IF YOU HAVE A PANIC ATTACK

Put a gap in your breathing. Go back to the section in this book about putting a gap in your breathing. Practice the exercise so you can use it the moment you feel panicky. Once you have any feelings of anxiety, panic, or worry, your breathing has already changed (you probably won't have noticed). So try to put a gap in your breathing as soon as possible so it returns to normal.

WHAT TO DO IN THE FUTURE

Once your Control Pause in above 40, you can reduce the amount of exercises you do per day. Keep an eye on the Control Pause making sure it remains high. These exercises 'reset' the breathing centre, so there is no need to do them every day for the rest of your life. However, if you have lung damage you may need to continue with them.

Do 6 SETS a day for a week then 5 SETS a day for a week. 4, the following week, etc, until you are down to 1 Set a day. If your Control Pause starts to drop, increase the amount of SETS you do. Do 1 SET a day for approximately 6 months. After that just do your Control Pause each morning to check your breathing. You may need to return to doing the exercises as before.

Tape your mouth every night for about 6 months then try without. Do this and monitor your Control Pause and pulse each night and the following morning for a week. Write down the results. If your Control Pause has gone down by morning, or your pulse up, your mouth will still be coming open. Try again with the tape for another 3 months.

38

A FEW FINAL WORDS

I hope you have found this book useful and have benefited from the exercises in it. I'd like to encourage you to continue to do the exercises after you've finished this book and to see how much more your health will improve. Hopefully you'll have noticed an improvement to your breathing already and you may have identified specific exercises that you'll want to do, when required, for the rest of your life. Reading this book, and doing the exercises in it, are the first few steps to good breathing and good health. I like to think of this as being a little like learning to drive: you have your lessons at the beginning, and then you take your test, and then the real learning begins over the following months and years as you deal with new situations.

If you want to learn more, I suggest you contact a Buteyko Practitioner or Breathing Retrainer. For more information search for 'Buteyko' on the internet.

Thanks for reading. I wish you well.

91800849R00093

Made in the USA
San Bernardino, CA
25 October 2018